Methylene Blue

Revolutionary Treatment for various
Diseases and Disorders

Craig Arnold

Table Of Contents

Introduction

Methylene blue is a heterocyclic aromatic molecule with Formula C16H18ClN3S. Since Heinrich Caro, a German scientist, originally synthesized it in 1876, it has been applied in several industrial, medical, and research settings. Deep blue, the chemical is easily recognized by its absorption spectra, which peak at approximately 600–700 nm in wavelength. Because Methylene Blue is so soluble in alcohol and water, it can be used as a stain and dye in histology and biology. Due to its distinct chemical makeup, it is also a useful treatment for a variety of diseases, especially those that include neurodegeneration or metabolic malfunction.

A chemical known for its versatility and revolutionary qualities, methylene blue (MB) has demonstrated considerable promise in treating a wide range of diseases. Because of its unique chemical and physical characteristics, MB has been utilized extensively in industry, science, and medicine since its discovery more than a century ago. The definition, historical background, broad applications, targeted therapeutic uses, safety concerns, and current research directions of MB are all summarized in this article.

The substance is a member of the phenothiazines class of organic compounds, which are distinguished by their planar structures and capacity to engage in redox processes.

Because of these characteristics, MB has become an invaluable tool for biological staining and imaging methods, which frequently involve using it to see cellular elements including mitochondria, lysosomes, and nuclei. Moreover, MB has proven to have strong antibacterial, anti-inflammatory, and antioxidant properties, broadening its potential uses beyond basic scientific studies.

Repurposing MB as a medicinal agent for a range of diseases has garnered more attention in recent years. According to studies, MB may protect against depression, stroke, and neurodegenerative diseases like Parkinson's and Alzheimer's disease. Moreover, MB has demonstrated encouraging outcomes in the fight against pathogenic agents such as bacteria, fungi, and parasites, providing fresh opportunities for the creation of innovative antimicrobials.

Even with these developments, questions still exist about the safety profile of MB, particularly when large doses or combinations with other drugs are taken. Therefore, to maximize its therapeutic potential while avoiding side effects, it is imperative to determine the ideal dose, time, and mode of administration.

The complex nature of MB will be examined in this review, along with its various uses and current efforts to fully realize its potential as a transformative therapy for various diseases and disorders. Through an exploration of the intricate relationships among MB's chemistry, biology, and pharmacology, we hope to illuminate this extraordinary molecule and stimulate more research into its plethora of fascinating applications.

Methylene Blue's past
The discovery of Methylene Blue (MB) by German chemist Heinrich Caro in 1876 began a lengthy and illustrious history that stretches back to the late 1800s. MB was first created as a textile dye, but it soon became well-known for its eye-catching blue hue and versatility as a substrate-binding agent. It was widely used in histology and microscopy once scientists realized in a matter of years how useful it might be as a biological stain.

One of the first known medical applications of MB was for the treatment of malaria in 1891 by Nobel winner and immunology and chemotherapy pioneer Paul Ehrlich. Surprisingly, MB showed remarkable effectiveness in lowering fever and getting rid of Plasmodium falciparum, the parasite that causes malignant tertian malaria. Building on this success, MB was used as a standard treatment for malaria until the mid-1900s, when more focused medicines became available.

More medicinal uses for MB were discovered by researchers over the twentieth century. For example, because it can cause a typical hypertensive crisis during provocative testing, it has become an essential diagnostic tool for pheochromocytoma, a rare tumor of the adrenal glands. Additionally, MB was a key player in the creation of cardiopulmonary resuscitation (CPR), acting as a vasodilator and an early oxygen carrier throughout the process.

The range of MB's indications grew together with our comprehension of its mechanisms of action. The World Health Organization's Model List of Essential Medicines still includes MB as a necessary ingredient, demonstrating the drug's ongoing importance in contemporary medicine. MB keeps expanding the frontiers of medical study and practice due to growing interest in its therapeutic potential for conditions ranging from neurodegeneration to cancer.

Methylene Blue's general usage and uses

Methylene Blue (MB) has been widely used in a variety of industries, including research, manufacturing, and medical, during the past century. Here, we go over a few of its most popular uses:

- Biological Stains and Tracers: MB is an effective stain and tracer in histology, cytology, and microbiology because it can form stable complexes with a variety of macromolecules. Because of its affinity for acidic substances, it can be used to identify organelles including the Golgi apparatus, mitochondria, and lysosomes, offering crucial information about the structure and operation of subcellular structures.

- Photodynamic Therapy: Methylene Blue (MB) is a key component of this technique, which uses light to activate photosensitizers and produce reactive oxygen species that can kill target cells. As MB reacts with visible light to produce singlet oxygen radicals that target malignant tissue specifically, it can be used to treat some forms of skin malignancies and precancers.

- Diagnostics: MB has proved helpful in the diagnosis of several diseases, especially those that impact the nervous system. Its tendency to cause hypertension in pheochromocytoma patients made this uncommon condition easier to diagnose. Analogously, methemoglobinemia—a condition marked by abnormal blood levels of methemoglobin—has also been tested for using MB.

- Cardiac Resuscitation: As was previously indicated, MB was crucial to the development of cardiopulmonary resuscitation (CPR). MB serves as a vasodilator and oxygen transporter during CPR techniques, enhancing oxygen delivery and perfusion to critical organs.

- Malaria Treatment: MB is still used as a backup treatment for drug-resistant types of Plasmodium spp., the protozoan parasites that cause malaria, even though it is no longer regarded as a frontline therapy. Remarkably, the WHO recommends artemisinin-based combinations, including MB, as the initial line of treatment for severe P. falciparum malaria.

- Antibacterial Agent: MB is a potentially appealing option for the development of novel antimicrobials due to its broad-spectrum antibacterial action against both Gram-positive and ----negative bacteria.

- Antiprotozoal Activity: MB exhibits effectiveness against several other protozoan pathogens, such as Giardia, Trypanosoma, and Leishmania donovani, indicating its wider relevance in treating neglected tropical diseases. This efficacy extends beyond malaria.

- Antiviral Effects: According to preliminary data, MB may have antiviral effects against a variety of viruses, including the influenza virus, herpes simplex virus, hepatitis C virus, and HIV. To determine its clinical utility assess its effectiveness when combined with conventional radiotherapy and chemotherapy techniques.

- Neurological Disorders: A growing body of research indicates that MB can be used to treat a variety of neurological conditions, from depression to Alzheimer's disease. By regulating nitric oxide signaling, inflammation, and oxidative stress, MB seems to have the potential to completely transform the way we treat crippling neuropsychiatric disorders.

These instances highlight the astounding range of uses for MB and its significance as a flexible and essential instrument in contemporary research and medicine.

Pharmacological Properties of Methylene Blue

Comprehending the pharmacologic characteristics of Methylene Blue (MB) is essential for recognizing its numerous uses in medical and scientific fields. We examine a few of its essential traits below:

- Chemical Structure and Properties: MB is made up of two benzene rings and a dimethylaniline moiety connected by azine bonds. Because of its flat, planar form, MB can effectively pass through lipophilic membranes and reach intracellular targets. It's interesting to note that, in contrast to other small molecules, MB primarily lives in its reduced state within cells, allowing for quick reduction-oxidation cycling and unique reactivity profiles.

- ADME (Absorption, Distribution, Metabolism, Excretion): After being administered orally or parenterally, MB enters the body quickly through the gastrointestinal tract or injection site, spreads across bodily fluids, and mostly concentrates inside erythrocytes. After that, it is primarily metabolized by the liver via the glucuronidation and sulfation conjugation pathways, and then it is excreted by the biliary system. About 10% of the overall elimination process is accomplished by renal clearance, suggesting that biliary obstruction or compromised liver function may result in prolonged exposure and a higher risk of toxicity.

- Mechanisms of Action: MB participates in several molecular interactions that support its pleiotropic effects. First of all, MB is a redox-active substance that easily alternates between its reduced (colorless) and oxidized (blue) forms. It does this by taking part in electron transfer reactions and replenishing NADPH, a vital cofactor in preserving cellular homeostasis. Second, MB suppresses several enzymes involved in signal transduction cascades, such as protein kinases, phosphodiesterases, and guanylate cyclase, which affects downstream effectors like cGMP, Ca^{2+}, and NO. Finally, reactive oxygen and nitrogen species produced during oxidative stress are quenched by MB by direct scavenging of free radicals. When taken as a whole, these behaviors have broad physiological effects that are pertinent to different disease conditions.

- Pharmacodynamics: Preclinical and clinical evidence indicates that MB exhibits concentration-dependent effects, with larger concentrations leading to cytotoxic or inhibitory effects and lower concentrations eliciting stimulatory responses. As a result, it is critical to adjust the dosage, frequency, and length of MB administration to maximize intended therapeutic advantages without sacrificing safety margins.

- Drug and Xenobiotic Interactions: Although MB has a long history of safe use, it interacts with a variety of medications and xenobiotics, thus careful thought should be given before administering them simultaneously. Concerning their potential for synergistic or additive interactions with MB, serotonergic drugs, sulfonamides, and antimalarials in particular deserve special mention. On the other hand, several drugs—like phenytoin, warfarin, and carbamazepine—may reduce the effectiveness of MB by speeding up its metabolism or raising its rates of excretion. Therefore, to reduce adverse effects, doctors should use caution when providing MB in addition to other drugs and thoroughly evaluate patient response.

Comprehending these pharmacological facets offers a valuable understanding of MB's adaptability and contributes to the logical development of experimental procedures intended to optimize its therapeutic benefits in various fields.

Properties And Structure Of Chemicals

A derivative of phenothiazine, methylene blue (MB) has the following molecular structure:

With a molecular weight of 319.85 g/mol, it is distinguished by a symmetrical, planar atom arrangement that increases lipophilicity and gives it stiffness. These characteristics make it easier for MB to cross cell membranes, which helps explain why it's found in so many different tissues and biofluids.

Among MB's noteworthy chemical characteristics are:

- Solubility: MB shows poor solubility in nonpolar solvents like ether and chloroform, but it dissolves easily in water, ethanol, and dimethyl sulfoxide (DMSO). The polar functional group's amido (-CONH2), sulfur (-SO3H), and amino (-NH2) substituents give it its hydrophilic nature.

- Redox (Reduction-Oxidation) Reactivity: MB's ability to participate in reversible one-electron transfer processes and switch between its reduced (colorless) leuco form and its oxidized (blue) form is one of its distinguishing characteristics. Because of this characteristic, MB is very well-suited to participate in redox chemistry, which affects a wide range of biological functions linked to signaling, detoxification, and energy production. Significantly, a lot of MB's medicinal uses are based on this duality, especially when restoring disturbed redox balance is necessary.

- Spectral Characteristics: Depending on its oxidation state, MB displays different optical characteristics. Oxidized MB has strong absorption maxima in the region of 610–670 nm in solution, which gives it its distinctive deep blue hue. However, these bands lose color when reduced because they move toward shorter wavelengths (about 300–400 nm). Thus, following alterations in MB's spectral profile provides an easy way to keep tabs on its redox condition in real-time, allowing evaluation of redox dynamics in living systems.

- Complex Formation: MB's ability to participate in ligand exchange processes and create coordination complexes with Lewis acids (like Al3+) or metal ions (like Fe2+, Cu2+, and Zn2+) is another noteworthy characteristic. These interactions affect not only the spectroscopic behavior and electronic structure of MB but also its reactivity and partitioning between aqueous and lipid phases, which in turn determines its overall behavior within the biological milieu.

All of these chemical characteristics provide MB with remarkable functionality, which explains much of its use as a research, therapeutic, and diagnostic probe in a variety of fields.

Mechanism of Action

Many of the ways that methylene blue (MB) works include changes to cellular redox balance, modulation of enzymes, and signaling pathways. Individual actions are contingent upon the particular environment and level of MB concentration, however, there are a few noteworthy kinds of action that are worth discussing here:

- Electron movement and Oxidoreductase Modulation: Due to its redox activity, MB takes part in electron shuttling reactions, which are activities that facilitate the movement of a single electron between donors and acceptors. By directly interacting with catalytic centers or indirectly altering cofactors necessary for enzyme function, it affects the activity of several oxidoreductases. Examples of enzymes that depend on MB for optimal function include complex IV (cytochrome c oxidase), succinate dehydrogenase, and NADH dehydrogenase in the respiratory chain.

- Guanylate Cyclase Inhibition: As a second messenger implicated in a variety of regulatory processes, soluble guanylate cyclase (sGC), an enzyme essential for converting GTP to cGMP, is inhibited by MB. MB inhibits nitric oxide (NO)-mediated activation by binding competitively to the ferrous iron core of sGC. This attenuates downstream signals linked to platelet aggregation, neuronal transmission, and vascular relaxation.

- Protein Kinase Regulation: cGMP is a necessary cofactor for the interaction of several protein kinases, most notably those belonging to the PKG family, with target proteins. As a result, PKG-dependent phosphorylation events are dampened by MB-induced reduction of sGC, disrupting signal transduction networks that are essential for cell migration, proliferation, and survival.

- Scavenging Free Radicals: MB neutralizes reactive oxygen and nitrogen species (ROS/RNS) and shields cells from oxidative damage because it is a strong antioxidant. By directly interacting with ROS/RNS, one can lower local concentrations and stop secondary reactions that could otherwise harm proteins, lipids, and DNA. Moreover, MB supports natural defense systems against oxidative stress by indirectly upregulating endogenous antioxidants.

- Metal Chelation: By noting heavy metals, MB creates insoluble precipitates that restrict their availability for later absorption by susceptible cell types. This characteristic takes on extra importance when an elevated metal load is linked to clinical symptoms, as in Wilson's disease, a hereditary condition characterized by dyshomeostasis of the copper ion channel.

- Membrane Permeabilization: High levels of MB encourage the outer and inner mitochondrial membranes to permeate, which causes the release of apoptogenic proteins and initiates programmed cell death. This behavior is usually unwanted in healthy cells, but it can be used as a tactic to eliminate transformed equivalents that carry faulty checkpoints or altered regulators controlling apoptosis.

All things considered, the mode of action of MB is reflective of its intrinsic malleability, permitting adjustment to a variety of settings and modification of different targets according to concentration gradients and temporal variations. Gaining a deeper comprehension of these complex relationships will enable us to fully utilize MB's therapeutic promise across a range of disease models.

Pharmaceutical Dynamics and Pharmacokinetics

It is essential to comprehend the pharmacokinetics and pharmacodynamics of Methylene Blue (MB) to properly recognize its clinical use and therapeutic index.

The term "pharmacokinetics" describes the progression of a drug's distribution, metabolism, excretion, and absorption over time in an organism. Important variables consist of:

Absorption:
When a drug is administered orally, it must first pass through the gastrointestinal (GI) tract before being absorbed into the bloodstream. This process involves several steps, including passage through the stomach, small intestine, and liver, where the drug may undergo metabolic changes known as pre-systemic metabolism or first-pass effect.

In the case of the drug called MB, it has been found to have significant pre-systemic metabolism and poor passive diffusion across the gut enterocytes, which are the cells lining the walls of the small intestine. As a result, only a small fraction of the drug can reach systemic circulation after oral administration, leading to low bioavailability.

Bioavailability refers to the extent and rate at which a drug becomes available in the systemic circulation after administration by a non-intravenous route, such as oral or subcutaneous injection. In other words, it measures how much of the drug reaches the target site of action and exerts its therapeutic effects. Low bioavailability means that a higher dose of the drug needs to be administered to achieve the desired clinical response, increasing the risk of adverse effects.

To overcome these limitations, parenteral methods of administration, such as intramuscular or subcutaneous injection, can be used instead. These routes allow the drug to bypass the GI tract and avoid pre-systemic metabolism, resulting in significantly larger plasma concentrations and faster onset of action compared to oral administration. Additionally, because the absorption and distribution of the drug are more predictable with parenteral administration, the effects of the drug can also be more reliably anticipated.

Distribution:
After a drug is absorbed from the GI tract or administered via another route, it enters the systemic circulation and begins to distribute throughout the body. The distribution of a drug depends on various factors, including its physiochemical properties, binding to plasma proteins, tissue perfusion, and membrane permeability.

MB is highly protein-bound, meaning that it predominantly circulates in the plasma attached to plasma proteins, primarily alpha-1-glycoprotein and albumin. Protein binding helps to facilitate the transport of drugs across cellular membranes, including those of the capillary endothelium, enabling them to easily access peripheral tissues.

The ability of a drug to cross the blood-brain barrier (BBB), a tightly regulated interface between the blood and brain tissues, is critical for central nervous system (CNS) activity. The BBB restricts the entry of most molecules, including drugs, into the CNS to maintain homeostasis and protect the delicate neural environment. However, some drugs, including MB, can cross the BBB, albeit to varying degrees.

Regional variations in blood flow rates and expression patterns of ATP-binding cassette (ABC) transporters, which actively pump drugs out of the brain, influence the degree to which MB penetrates the BBB. Generally speaking, regions of the brain with lower blood flow rates and decreased expression of ABC transporters exhibit greater accumulation of MB. Once inside the CNS, MB achieves relatively low levels in the cerebrospinal fluid (CSF). Specifically, CSF levels of MB typically range from 10-30% of corresponding plasma values. Nonetheless, even modest increases in CNS exposure can produce meaningful therapeutic responses.

Metabolism:
Metabolism is a crucial step in the disposition of xenobiotics, including drugs, in the human body. Xenobiotic metabolizing enzymes transform lipophilic compounds into more polar, water-soluble forms, facilitating their elimination from the body. Drug metabolism occurs primarily in the liver, although extrahepatic metabolism also plays a role in some cases.

MB undergoes extensive phase II metabolism, which involves the addition of functional groups such as glucuronic acid, sulfuric acid, or acetic acid to enhance the compound's polarity and solubility. Phase II reactions generally follow phase I reactions, which involve oxidative, reductive, or hydrolytic modifications of the parent compound. However, since MB does not undergo any appreciable phase I metabolism, it proceeds directly to phase II metabolism.

Glucuronidation represents the major pathway for MB metabolism, accounting for over 95% of total clearance. Two distinct glucuronide products are formed - monoglucuronide and diglucuronide - reflecting the attachment of one or two glucuronic acid moieties, respectively. Both metabolites are ultimately eliminated via urinary excretion.

Ring hydroxylation and sulfate conjugation represent minor metabolic pathways for MB, contributing less than 5% of total clearance. Hydroxylation introduces a polar group onto the aromatic ring structure, promoting water solubility and subsequent renal elimination. Sulfate conjugation entails the addition of a sulfuryl (-SO4) group, enhancing the overall charge and polarity of the compound. Together, these minor metabolic pathways contribute to the complete elimination of MB from the body.

Interindividual variability in drug-metabolizing enzyme activity can substantially impact the metabolism and elimination of xenobiotics, potentially affecting drug efficacy and toxicity profiles. Factors influencing enzyme activity include genetic variation, age, sex, diet, disease state, and concomitant medication usage. Understanding the complex interplay between these variables and drug metabolism enables personalized medicine approaches aimed at optimizing therapy outcomes while minimizing adverse events.

Excretion:

Excretion is the final step in the journey of a drug within the body. Following metabolism, the metabolites and unchanged drugs are eliminated from the body mainly through either urine or feces, depending on the physicochemical properties of the drug and its metabolites.

As mentioned earlier, MB undergoes extensive phase II metabolism, generating derivatives of mono- and bis-glucuronides. Unaltered MB and its metabolites are largely eliminated in the urine, representing approximately 85-90% of the total dose administered. Only trace quantities of MB or its metabolites appear in the feces.

A portion of the filtered metabolites and unaltered drug may be subject to reabsorption in the renal tubules, thereby reducing the amount excreted in the urine. This phenomenon, termed tubular reabsorption, contributes to the overall pharmacokinetics of the drug. However, the majority of MB and its metabolites do not undergo tubular reabsorption due to their high polarity.

Some metabolites and unaltered drugs may undergo enterohepatic recycling, involving secretion into the bile, followed by deconjugation in the intestines by bacterial enzymes, then reabsorption back into the circulation. Enterohepatic cycling can prolong the duration of drug action; however, it does not play a substantial role in MB's elimination.

Clearance refers to the volume of plasma cleared of a drug per unit of time, often expressed as mL/min or L/hr. Creatinine clearance is a commonly used measure of renal function, reflecting the filtration capacity of the kidneys. Importantly, the clearance of many drugs correlates closely with creatinine clearance, indicating that individuals with impaired renal function may require dose adjustments to prevent excessive drug accumulation and related toxicities.

Since MB's clearance follows linear kinetics relative to creatinine clearance, reductions in renal function can lead to increased drug exposure. Consequently, clinicians may need to modify the dosage of MB in patients with compromised renal function to ensure safe and effective treatment outcomes. Monitoring serum creatinine levels and estimated creatinine clearance can assist healthcare providers in making informed decisions about appropriate dosing strategies in patients receiving MB therapy.

The link between drug concentration and the observed effect is known as pharmacodynamics, and it is represented by conventional sigmoidal dose-response curves that characterize agonists, antagonists, or inverse agonists. Important components include:

Receptor Occupancy Theory:
MB binds to target proteins in a competitive antagonistic manner, preventing natural ligands from attaching and so

upsetting downstream signaling cascades. As MB and endogenous agonists compete, equilibrium is shifted toward favorable displacement in a way that is correlated with relative abundance and affinity constants.

Signal Transduction Pathways:
Depending on the activated pathways and the net sum of positive vs negative inputs, the downstream effects of receptor occupation might differ significantly. For instance, soluble guanylate cyclase is blocked by MB-mediated inhibition, which reduces the production of cGMP and blunts the effects of nitric oxide (NO), which is responsible for vasodilation, platelet inhibition, and neuronal excitement.

Temporal Considerations:
Residence half-life and turnover rate within active sites have a significant impact on time-dependent kinetics, which in turn affects MB's overall efficacy. Decreased extracellular levels can still cause interference with slow off-rate constants, maintaining desired effects even with brief exposures.

Concentration Thresholds:
MB moves from hostility to direct agonism above a specific threshold, causing opposite results from what was originally intended. It becomes necessary to titrate carefully

and monitor closely to maintain within optimal limits free of undesirable side effects.

In the end, combining pharmacokinetic and pharmacodynamic principles provides a thorough framework for logically-based dosage plans catered to specific requirements, ensuring maximum benefit moderated by tolerable limits and safety considerations.

Therapeutic Applications of Methylene Blue

Because of its diverse method of action, Methylene Blue (MB) has a broad range of therapeutic uses. Among the recognized uses are:

- Antimalarial Therapy: MB, which acts as a redox cycler to promote hemozoin synthesis, was formerly the main drug used to treat malaria brought on by Plasmodium falciparum infection. As of right now, the World Health Organization includes it in its list of recommended artemisinin-based combination therapy.

- Methemoglobinemia Correction: Deficits in nicotinamide adenine dinucleotide phosphate (NADPH)-dependent reductase activity that underlie acquired or hereditary types of methemoglobinemia are effectively addressed by MB, restoring methemoglobin to normal hemoglobin.

- Neuroprotection: MB protects delicate neuronal circuits against degenerative attacks seen in ischemic strokes, traumatic brain traumas, and Parkinson's disease by maintaining mitochondrial integrity, increasing ATP generation, and reducing excitotoxicity.

- Reduction of Depression Symptoms: In patients who are not responding to therapy, low-dose MB increases noradrenergic and dopaminergic tone, reducing depression symptoms. The processes that have been proposed center on increased recycling of monoamines and decreased oxidative stress caused by stronger antioxidant defenses.

- Parasitic Disease Management: By affecting the viability, morphology, or invasiveness of parasites, MB also successfully fights off giardiasis, cryptosporidiosis, leishmaniasis, Chagas disease, babesiosis, and trypanosomiasis.

- Cardiovascular Support: MB helps cases of congestive heart failure or hypotensive episodes by relaxing smooth muscles and bolstering contractility. It also decreases the degree of pulmonary edema and enhances right ventricular function after heart surgery.

- Mitochondrial Dysfunction Rectification: MB corrects the aging-related or disease-related impairments to mitochondrial energetics and architecture, including sepsis, diabetes, and chronic obstructive pulmonary disease (COPD).

- Antimicrobial Utility: Because of its broad-spectrum bacteriostatic qualities, MB can be used for catheter coatings, topical wound care, and periodontal therapy. There are synergistic relationships between conventional antibiotics and other drugs, suggesting possible approaches to address the growing problem of resistance.

- Oncology Adjuvant: New research suggests that MB increases therapeutic windows, reduces collateral harm to neighboring normal tissues, and sensitizes cancerous cells to ionizing radiation and chemotherapy.

- Experimental Medicine Toolbox: MB is a critical marker that is widely used in scientific research to trace neural circuitry, measure oxygen tension, quantify autofluorescence, calibrate optogenetic instruments, and validate assays that rely on flavoprotein autofluorescence, among other uses.

Methylene Blue has remarkable adaptability across several therapeutic domains, mostly attributed to its strong redox properties, adjustable pharmacokinetics, and flexible pharmacodynamics. Additional research is underway to uncover novel applications for this age-old substance that is still amazingly relevant.

Methemoglobinemia Treatment

Elevated levels of methemoglobin (MetHb), a modified type of hemoglobin that is ineffective in carrying oxygen, are the hallmarks of methemoglobinemia. Adult human blood typically has less than 1% MetHb, but significant increases impair the oxygen delivery to tissues, resulting in symptoms including cyanosis, exhaustion, headaches, dyspnea, and potentially fatal consequences if ignored. MetHb-associated problems fall into two main categories: acquired and congenital (inherited). Congenital variations result from genetic mutations that code for defective enzymes, primarily cytochrome b5 reductase and diaphorase I, which are responsible for converting MetHb back to functional hemoglobin. Claimed cases can be traced back to external assaults or medications that cause oxidative stress greater than the body's natural antioxidant reserves, overriding the body's ability to compensate. Nitrites, nitrates, derivatives of aniline, phenols, benzenes, and several medications (including lidocaine, prilocaine, and dapsone) are common causes.

Ascorbic acid, methylene blue (MB), or hyperbaric oxygen (HBO) therapy were the usual preferred management methods. Among them, MB is unique in that it quickly resolves symptoms and is less expensive than other options. In contrast, ascorbic acid requires higher cumulative dosages, exhibits inconsistent efficiency, and performs less well than MB in terms of both the rate and extent of improvement. Hyperbaric oxygen has little practical application outside of certain conditions due to the need for specialist facilities, longer periods, and logistical challenges. Therefore, MB becomes the recommended option for the treatment of methemoglobinemia.

Mechanistically, MB functions as an electron donor, supplying MetHb reductase, an enzyme that is dependent on NADPH to convert MetHb to functional hemoglobin. Minutes after injection, there are rapid decreases that are followed by prompt symptom alleviation, a return to normal oxygen saturation, and a decline in MetHb fractions below dangerous values. Intravenous administration of 1-2 mg/kg body weight over five minutes is the standard starting dose. This can be repeated every hour if necessary until stability occurs. Keeping an eye on serial measures guarantees proper management, timely action, and a steer clear of dangerously low MetHb percentages that might cause hemolysis.

Despite its benefits, MB has several drawbacks that should be noted. In particular, those with glucose-6-phosphate dehydrogenase (G6PD) impairment need to be excluded from pretreatment screening since they are more susceptible to hemolytic crises brought on by MB-mediated MetHb decrease. Similarly, because of the potential for teratogenic effects and unknown fetal tolerance, pregnant women and nursing mothers should be handled with caution. Lastly, allergic reactions are an additional issue that needs attention before starting therapy.

All things considered, MB is a proven treatment for methemoglobinemia that combines effectiveness, affordability, and ease of administration. However, wise use requires awareness of potential hazards to get the best results while avoiding untoward situations.

Neuroprotective Properties

Growing research demonstrates that methylene blue (MB) multifactorial mechanism of action contributes to its neuroprotective effectiveness against a range of neurological diseases. The main processes include increased ATP production, reduced excitotoxicity, reduced inflammation, and strengthened antioxidant defenses, all of which contribute to the lifetime of neurons under adverse microenvironments. MB's neuroprotective properties are beneficial for several notable ailments, including:

Ischemic Stroke
Ischemia, which is partially caused by calcium excess and the ensuing glutamatergic excitotoxicity, results in permanent neuronal death. MB fights these harmful processes by doing the following:

1 Guanylate cyclase inhibition, which prevents cerebral edema and prevents vasodilation mediated by cyclic guanosine monophosphate (cGMP).

2 Blockade of protein kinase G (PKG), which limits deleterious phosphorylation cascades started by cGMP.

3 Improving Complex IV, increasing ATP supply, and reducing energy shortage.

4 NMDA receptor antagonistic action, preventing over-influx of calcium and subsequent depolarization of the cell.

Traumatic Brain Injury (TBI):
TBI causes significant structural damage to impacted areas, leading to a loss of neurological function. MB combats the harm caused by TBI via:

1 Enhanced mitochondrial performance, preventing apoptosis and boosting energy stores.

2 Reduced activity of matrix metallopeptidase-9 (MMP-9), which limits neuroinflammation and moderates the breakdown of the blood-brain barrier.

Reduced generation of reactive oxygen species (ROS), reducing the oxidative stress placed on delicate tissues.

Parkinson's Disease
PD is characterized by a slow and steady degeneration of dopaminergic neurons in the substantia nigra pars compacta, which leads to cognitive dysfunction and movement deficits. MB lessens the symptoms of PD by:

1. Increased tyrosine hydroxylase activity, which restores depleted dopamine levels.

2 Decreased alpha-synuclein aggregation, which hinders the development and spread of Lewy bodies.

3. Increased mitochondrial toughness, supporting strained organelles that are prone to breaking.

Alzheimer's disease (AD):
AD is characterized by tau tangle and beta-amyloid plaque buildups, which lead to memory loss, language problems, and executive dysfunctions. MB responds to AD characteristics by:

1 Decreased beta-amyloid fibrillization, which inhibits the formation of misfolded peptides and the resulting neurotoxicity.

2 Threw off the tau hyperphosphorylation, which stopped the instability of microtubules and the disruption of axonal transport.

3. Increased antioxidant capability, which reduces oxidative stress and buffers redox imbalance.

Multiple sclerosis
Myelin sheaths that envelop nerve fibers are destroyed by the immune system in multiple sclerosis (MS), resulting in conduction defects and neurological impairment. MB slows the course of MS by:

1. Modified the polarization of CD4+ T-cells, skewing the proportion of helper T-cell subsets away from the pathogenic Th1 and Th17 phenotypes.

2. Suppressed astrogliosis, which prevents the reactive gliosis that causes lesions to enlarge and scars to develop.

3 Blood-brain barrier integrity was restored, reducing the impact of an autoimmune assault on components of the central nervous system.

Methylene blue has several diverse neuroprotective properties that make it a useful treatment for a range of neurological conditions. However, to confirm these promising preclinical findings and convert them into real therapeutic benefits for affected patients, prospective randomized controlled studies are still necessary.

Alzheimer's disease

Alzheimer's disease (AD) is a neurological disease that worsens with time and is marked by behavioral abnormalities, memory loss, and cognitive impairment. Millions of people are impacted globally, and both families and healthcare systems are severely burdened. Regretfully, current therapies do nothing more than momentarily reduce symptoms without stopping or turning back the course of the disease. It is therefore critically necessary to develop novel treatment approaches that target underlying diseases. Let's introduce methylene blue (MB), a substance whose potential to lessen AD-associated neuropathology is becoming more widely acknowledged.

The three main processes behind MB's alleged benefits in AD are as follows:
Anti-amyloidogenic activity: Alzheimer's disease (AD) is characterized by senile plaques, which are formed when amyloid-beta (Aβ) peptides combine into insoluble fibrils. According to in vitro research, MB lessens neurotoxicity by disassembling produced fibrils and preventing Aβ fibrillization. Furthermore, after MB treatment, animal models show decreased amyloidosis and enhanced cognition.

Characteristics of antioxidants: In AD, oxidative stress, which is fueled by reactive oxygen species (ROS), plays a major role in the destruction of neurons. Because of its role as an electron transporter, MB facilitates electron transfer and, as a result, neutralizes ROS and reduces oxidative damage.

Mitochondrial protection: Neuronal survival is negatively impacted by mitochondrial dysfunction and energy shortages that accompany AD. MB promotes overall mitochondrial health and function by improving mitochondrial respiration, increasing ATP generation, and preventing oxidative damage.

Even with these encouraging results in the lab, translational success has been difficult to achieve. Mild increases in global function and cognition were seen in phase II clinical studies; however, these advantages were not supported in further stages. The current emphasis of the research is on reformulating MB into prodrugs or nanoparticles to improve bioavailability and perhaps improve blood-brain barrier penetration. On the other hand, combination therapy combining MB with licensed AD drugs may have beneficial benefits that warrant investigation.

Methylene blue is a strong contender in the search for new therapies for AD. Its diverse activities have great potential, but achieving this will need improved formulations and tactical partnerships that connect preclinical discoveries with clinical applications.

Parkinson's disease

In the substantia nigra pars compacta area of the midbrain, dopaminergic neurons gradually disappear in Parkinson's disease (PD), a neurodegenerative condition. The patient's quality of life is significantly impacted by this degeneration, which causes motor deficits, tremors, stiffness, and postural instability. Current therapies do not stop or reverse the course of the disease; instead, they aim to imitate or replace missing dopamine. Because of its pleiotropic properties, methylene blue (MB) has attracted interest as a possible possibility for novel treatment techniques that address underlying diseases.

The potential advantages of MB for Parkinson's disease can be explained by four main mechanisms:

Mitochondrial protection: Parkinson's disease (PD) is highly linked to mitochondrial malfunction, which is a factor in the death of neurons. MB promotes overall mitochondrial health and function by improving mitochondrial respiration, increasing ATP generation, and preventing oxidative damage.

Antioxidant properties: Elevated ROS and oxidative stress are important in the pathophysiology of Parkinson's disease. Because of its role as an electron transporter, MB facilitates electron transfer and, as a result, neutralizes ROS and reduces oxidative damage.

Activation of tyrosine hydroxylase: Tyrosine hydroxylase (TH) is an enzyme that limits the pace at which dopamine is synthesized. It has been demonstrated that MB increases TH activity, which raises dopamine levels and may help with motor symptom relief.

Neuroprotection: The development of Lewy bodies and the aggregation of alpha-synuclein are two important aspects of Parkinson's disease. MB may have neuroprotective effects by preventing toxicity and reducing alpha-synuclein aggregation, according to reports.

These suggested pathways are supported by preclinical research using in vitro assays and animal models, which show that MB therapy improves motor function, decreases neurodegeneration, and reduces alpha-synuclein aggregation. It has been challenging to successfully translate these discoveries into clinical studies, though. Open-label pilot studies were promising at first, but double-blind placebo-controlled trials were unable to consistently show advantages. More research is necessary since more recently, altered formulations of MB, such as L-DOPA-linked MB, have demonstrated positive outcomes in preclinical investigations.

However, because of its variety of effects, methylene blue is a viable option for treating Parkinson's disease. However, to fully realize its promise, it will need to bridge the gap between preclinical discoveries and concrete therapeutic advantages for patients through well-designed clinical trials, strategic partnerships, and optimized formulations.

Anxiety and Depression

Anxiety disorders and major depressive disorder (MDD) are common mental health issues that impact millions of people globally. Monoaminergic neurotransmission, notably that of dopamine, norepinephrine, and serotonin, is the major target of current therapy. These methods, however, have limited effectiveness and could have negative consequences. The chemical methylene blue (MB), with a variety of pharmacological characteristics, has gained attention as a possible treatment option for mood disorders because of its capacity to regulate monoaminergic neurotransmitters, as well as its antioxidant and neuroprotective qualities.

The potential benefits of MB for MDD and anxiety disorders can be explained by several mechanisms:

Monoaminergic modulation: MB blocks the action of the enzyme monoamine oxidase A (MAO-A), which is in charge of hydrolyzing dopamine, norepinephrine, and serotonin. MB improves the availability of these neurotransmitters by suppressing MAO-A, which may lessen feelings of anxiety and depression.

Two characteristics of antioxidants: Oxidative stress is essential to the pathogenesis of anxiety disorders and Major Depressive Disorder. As an electron carrier, MB facilitates the flow of electrons and, as a result, neutralizes reactive oxygen species (ROS) and reduces oxidative damage.

Neuroprotection: The pathophysiology of anxiety disorders and MDD is linked to glutamatergic excitotoxicity and neuroinflammation. It has been demonstrated that MB offers possible neuroprotective advantages by reducing neuroinflammation and guarding against glutamate-induced damage.

BDNF Gene Expression: The development, survival, and synaptic plasticity of neurons depend on brain-derived neurotrophic factor (BDNF). Anxiety disorders and Major Depressive Disorder are linked to decreased BDNF levels. According to reports, MB increases the expression of the BDNF gene, which promotes neuroplasticity and may lessen symptoms of anxiety and depression.

These suggested pathways are supported by preclinical research using in vitro tests and animal models, which show that MB therapy improves emotional behaviors, decreases neurodegeneration, and raises BDNF levels. Few clinical trials have examined the effectiveness of MB in treating mood disorders; the findings have been inconsistent. While open-label research has yielded encouraging results, double-blind, placebo-controlled experiments have yielded conflicting results. To treat MDD and anxiety disorders, more study is required to discover the best MB dose, formulation, and mode of administration.

Because of its variety of effects, methylene blue shows promise as a treatment for anxiety disorders and major depressive diseases. Its small window of efficacy to toxicity means that, to fully realize its promise, well-planned clinical studies and more research into refining its therapeutic window are necessary. Patients with mood disorders may benefit from complementary advantages and better overall results if MB is used with current therapy.

Traumatic Brain Injury and Stroke

Globally, stroke and traumatic brain injury (TBI) are major causes of morbidity and mortality. Different degrees of brain impairments are caused by these diseases, and survivors frequently have lifetime problems. Due to the intricacy of these diseases, multipronged therapy techniques are necessary, and because of their various pharmacological characteristics, methylene blue (MB) has emerged as a possible possibility.

The potential benefits of MB for stroke and traumatic brain injury can be explained by many mechanisms:

Mitochondrial Dysfunction: Dysfunction of the mitochondria, which leads to neuronal death, is linked to stroke and traumatic brain injury. MB promotes overall mitochondrial health and function by improving mitochondrial respiration, increasing ATP generation, and preventing oxidative damage.

Antioxidant qualities: Elevated ROS and oxidative stress are key players in the pathophysiology of stroke and traumatic brain injury. As an electron carrier, MB facilitates the flow of electrons and, as a result, neutralizes reactive oxygen species (ROS) and reduces oxidative damage.

Neuroprotection: The pathogenesis of TBI and stroke involves excitotoxicity, neuroinflammation, and apoptosis. MB may have neuroprotective effects since it has been demonstrated to guard against glutamate-induced toxicity, lessen neuroinflammation, and prevent apoptosis.

Enhancement of cerebral blood flow: Traumatic brain injury and stroke frequently lead to decreased cerebral blood flow, which exacerbates ischemia damage. It has been shown that MB increases blood flow and dilates cerebral arteries, which may lessen ischemia damage.

These suggested pathways are supported by preclinical research using in vitro assays and animal models, which show that MB therapy improves neurological outcomes, reduces infarct sizes, and reduces neuroinflammation. It has been challenging to successfully use these findings in clinical studies, though. Although small pilot studies have suggested some advantages, large-scale randomized controlled trials have not yet proved that MB is beneficial for TBI or stroke.

Methylene blue's diverse range of activities makes it a potentially effective treatment option for stroke and traumatic brain injury. However, to fully realize its promise, it will need to bridge the gap between preclinical discoveries and concrete therapeutic advantages for patients through well-designed clinical trials, strategic partnerships, and optimized formulations. For stroke and traumatic brain injury survivors, adding MB to current therapies or using it as an adjuvant therapy may offer supplementary advantages and enhance overall results.

Antimicrobial Qualities

The antimicrobial effects of methylene blue (MB) have been demonstrated against a range of microorganisms, such as fungi, bacteria, and parasites. Numerous mechanisms are responsible for its antimicrobial action, such as the production of reactive oxygen species (ROS), rupturing bacterial membranes, suppressing bacterial enzymes, and interfering with quorum sensing.

Generation of ROS: MB can produce ROS, including hydroxyl radicals, hydrogen peroxide, and superoxide anion, which harm bacterial membranes, cell walls, and DNA and ultimately cause bacterial death.

Bacterial membrane disruption: MB can implant itself into bacterial membranes, rupturing their integrity and allowing intracellular contents to escape, which eventually results in bacterial death.

Inhibition of bacterial enzymes: It has been demonstrated that MB inhibits bacterial enzymes necessary for DNA replication and repair, including bacterial topoisomerases.

Quorum sensing interference: Bacteria use quorum sensing as a communication mechanism to coordinate group actions including the production of biofilms and the release of virulence factors. It has been demonstrated that MB inhibits quorum sensing, which lowers bacterial pathogenicity and inhibits the production of biofilms.

Acinetobacter baumannii, Pseudomonas aeruginosa, Escherichia coli, Klebsiella pneumoniae, methicillin-resistant Staphylococcus aureus (MRSA), vancomycin-resistant Enterococci (VRE), and other gram-positive and gram-negative bacteria have all been shown to be susceptible to the antimicrobial action of MB. Furthermore, it has been shown that MB is effective against parasites like Plasmodium falciparum, the cause of malaria, and fungal infections like Candida albicans.

The practical application of MB as an antibacterial agent is restricted because of problems with its solubility, stability, and possible toxicity at higher doses, despite its promising antimicrobial capabilities. However, the creation of MB-loaded liposomes and nanoparticles has been made possible by recent developments in drug delivery technologies and nanotechnology, which may enhance the medication's stability, safety, and bioavailability. Given the current state of antibiotic resistance and the pressing need for new antimicrobial treatments, these advancements provide the potential for repurposing MB as a potent antimicrobial agent.

Methylene blue demonstrates strong antibacterial qualities against a range of microbes via several methods. Novel avenues for its therapeutic application as an antibacterial agent have been made possible by developments in drug delivery methods and nanotechnology, offering promise for the treatment of microbial diseases and drug-resistant infections alike.

Effects Against Cancer

Recent years have seen a major increase in interest in methylene blue (MB) due to possible anti-cancer properties. Numerous investigations into the mechanisms of action of MB have revealed that, among other anti-cancer effects, it can restrict angiogenesis, cause apoptosis, and decrease the growth of cancer cells.

- Apoptosis induction: It has been demonstrated that MB may cause apoptosis in a variety of cancer cell lines, including those from the colon, lung, breast, prostate, and pancreas. It accomplishes this by blocking anti-apoptotic proteins like Bcl-2 and surviving and activating pro-apoptotic proteins like Bak, Bax, and caspases.

- Cell cycle arrest: By causing cancer cells to enter a cell cycle arrest, MB can stop the cells from proliferating. It does this by adjusting the expression and function of many cell cycle regulators, including CDK inhibitors, cyclins, and cyclin-dependent kinases (CDKs).

- inhibition of angiogenesis: Tumor development and metastasis depend on angiogenesis, the creation of new blood vessels. It has been shown that MB inhibits angiogenesis by upregulating anti-angiogenic factors such as thrombospondin-1 and downregulating pro-angiogenic factors like VEGF and HIF-1α.

- Inhibition of invasion and metastasis: By regulating the production and activity of matrix metalloproteinases (MMPs), which break down the extracellular matrix and aid in the spread of cancer cells, MB has been demonstrated to reduce the invasion and metastasis of cancer cells.

- Chemosensitization: MB can increase cancer cells' sensitivity to chemotherapeutic drugs, increasing their susceptibility to apoptosis brought on by therapy. It is believed that MB's capacity to regulate drug efflux pump function, obstruct DNA repair mechanisms, and increase oxidative stress in cancer cells is the cause of this chemosensitization effect.

- Even though these results are encouraging, more investigation is required to completely grasp MB's potential as an anti-cancer drug. Preliminary findings from clinical trials assessing MB's safety and effectiveness in cancer patients suggest that it could be a useful addition to conventional chemotherapy treatments that are well-tolerated. In the end, the discovery of MB as an anti-cancer drug could offer a fresh and useful supplement to the array of cancer treatments available today.

Methylene blue demonstrates strong anti-cancer properties via several pathways, such as triggering apoptosis, stopping the cell cycle, preventing angiogenesis, preventing invasion and metastasis, and causing chemosensitization. Its safety and effectiveness in cancer patients are being investigated in ongoing clinical trials; if successful, it might be a useful supplement to currently available cancer treatments.

Other Treatment

Methylene blue (MB) has demonstrated therapeutic potential in several additional areas in addition to treating methemoglobinemia, neurological diseases, anxiety and depression disorders, stroke and traumatic brain damage, antimicrobial qualities, and anti-cancer activities.

- Malaria: The World Health Organization recommends using artemisinin-based combination treatments (ACTs) to treat uncomplicated Plasmodium falciparum malaria. MB has been used historically as an antimalarial drug. By blocking the parasite's mitochondrial electron transport chain, MB causes reactive oxygen species to be produced, which in turn causes the parasite to die.

- Drug-induced methemoglobinemia: Nitrates, sulfonamides, and aniline dyes are some examples of drugs that can cause drug-induced methemoglobinemia. MB has been used to treat this condition with efficacy. Through the reduction of methemoglobin to hemoglobin, MB aids in the restoration of normal red blood cell activity.

- Congenital methemoglobinemia: Chronically high amounts of methemoglobin can result from several genetic diseases, including hemoglobin M disease and cytochrome b5 reductase deficiency. By lowering methemoglobin levels and easing hypoxia-related symptoms, MB can aid in the management of several diseases.

- Opthalmology: MB has been used in ophthalmology for several purposes, including treating retinitis pigmentosa, a hereditary eye disease marked by gradual vision loss, and coloring contact lens ulcers. Although the precise processes behind MB's advantages for the eyes remain mostly unclear, it is thought that both its antioxidant qualities and its capacity to alter mitochondrial activity contribute to its medicinal effects.

- Fungal infections: Aspergillus fumigatus, Candida albicans, and Cryptococcus neoformans are only a few of the fungal species against which MB has shown antifungal action. Its capacity to damage fungal cell membranes and prevent ergosterol biosynthesis—a critical component of fungal cell membranes—is assumed to be the source of its antifungal effect.

- Wound healing: It has been demonstrated that topical use of MB accelerates the healing of pressure ulcers, venous leg ulcers, and diabetic foot ulcers. Although the exact processes underpinning MB's ability to heal wounds are not fully known, it is believed that the drug's antibacterial, anti-inflammatory, and pro-angiogenic characteristics play a role.

Safety and Toxicity of Methylene Blue

Side Effects and Contraindications

Side Effects

Although methylene blue (MB) has a modest toxicity profile, it can nonetheless have negative effects in certain groups or at large dosages. Gastrointestinal upset, headaches, dizziness, and blue-green staining of body fluids such as perspiration, feces, and urine are common adverse effects of MB. Usually minor and self-limiting, these side effects go away quickly when the medication is stopped.

Irregular or combined usage of MB with some drugs may result in more severe side effects. For instance, MB is a mild monoamine oxidase inhibitor (MAOI) that might cause serotonin syndrome when used with other serotonergic medications or selective serotonin reuptake inhibitors (SSRIs). The symptoms of serotonin syndrome, which can be fatal, include agitation, disorientation, shivering, sweating, diarrhea, tachycardia, hypertension, stiffness in the muscles, and hyperreflexia. Healthcare professionals should regularly monitor patients receiving MB treatment for indications of serotonin syndrome and should inform patients about the hazards of using MB with other drugs.

Hemolysis in patients with a documented impairment of glucose-6-phosphate dehydrogenase (G6PD) is another possible side effect of MB. A hereditary condition called

G6PD deficiency impairs red blood cells' capacity to withstand oxidative stress. In some people, MB may lead to oxidative damage to red blood cells, which can result in hemolysis and potentially fatal anemia. In patients with a known G6PD deficiency, MB should be avoided.

Finally, because MB may pass the placenta and has been demonstrated to impact fetal development in animals, it should be taken cautiously during pregnancy. Pregnant women should only take MB if the possible benefits outweigh the dangers, as its safety in human pregnancy has not been thoroughly demonstrated.

Restrictions
The following are a few situations in which using MB is not appropriate:
- Known sensitivity to MB or any of its constituents
- G6PD insufficiency
- severe liver or kidney damage
- Usage of drugs that are serotonergic (because serotonin syndrome is a concern)
- Porphyria (since it may intensify symptoms of the condition)
- pregnancy (because of the possible danger to the fetus)

Before prescribing MB to patients, healthcare professionals should check for these contraindications. They should also keep a close eye out for any evidence of side effects in patients getting MB medication. The hazards connected with MB use can be reduced, and the best possible outcomes for patients can be guaranteed, with early identification and care.

Drug Interactions

Methylene blue (MB) has the potential to cause major side effects when it interacts with certain pharmaceutical types. Healthcare professionals have to be aware of these interactions and take precautions against the hazards that come with using MB.

Inhibitors of Monoamine Oxidase (MAOIs)
Due to its poor MAOI activity, MB can prevent monoamines including dopamine, serotonin, and norepinephrine from being broken down. MB may raise the risk of serotonin syndrome, a potentially fatal disease marked by symptoms including agitation, disorientation, shivering, sweating, diarrhea, tachycardia, hypertension, muscular stiffness, and hyperreflexia, when used with other MAOIs or serotonergic drugs. Healthcare professionals should regularly monitor patients receiving MB treatment for indications of serotonin syndrome and should inform patients about the hazards of using MB with other drugs.

QT-Prolonging Drugs

The QT interval, a gauge of the heart's electrical activity, can be extended by MB. MB may raise the risk of serious arrhythmias such as torsades de pointes when used with other drugs that also lengthen the QT interval. Healthcare professionals should be aware of this risk and, if at all feasible, refrain from providing MB in conjunction with other drugs that prolong QT. Patients who require co-administration should be closely watched for any indications of arrhythmias.

Medicines that lower blood pressure
MB may lower blood pressure, especially when taken in large quantities. When used with other antihypertensive drugs, MB may raise the risk of orthostatic hypotension, which is a transient dip in blood pressure that can cause fractures, disorientation, and falls. To reduce the risk of orthostatic hypotension, healthcare professionals should be aware of this risk and counsel patients to get up carefully from a sitting or lying posture.

Drugs that are anticoagulant and antiplatelet
A higher risk of bleeding can result from MB's interference with platelet function. MB may raise the risk of bleeding problems when used with other anticoagulants or antiplatelet drugs. Healthcare professionals should be aware of this risk and keep a watchful eye out for any bleeding symptoms in patients getting MB treatment.

Additional Exchanges

The following other drugs may also interact with MB:

- Inducers or inhibitors of the cytochrome P450 enzyme, which may impact the metabolism and clearance of MB
- Nitrates may combine with MB to form methylene blue nitrite, which may have the ability to constrict blood vessels in the lungs.
- Metoclopramide can reduce the bioavailability and absorption of MB.

Administration & Dosage

The indication being treated, the patient's age and weight, and the mode of administration all influence the proper methylene blue (MB) dose and administration. When prescribing MB, medical professionals have to adhere to established protocols and recommendations.

Based on Indication Dosage
Methemoglobinemia

The usual first intravenous dosage of MB for the treatment of methemoglobinemia is 1-2 mg/kg body weight given gradually over a few minutes. The dosage can be repeated every 30 to 60 minutes, depending on methemoglobin levels and clinical response. The highest dosage that is advised is 7 mg/kg of body weight.

Neuro Defense

MB has been investigated for its neuroprotective properties in neurological diseases at dosages ranging from 5 mg/kg body weight to 20 mg/kg body weight, either orally or intravenously. The optimum course of action requires more investigation as the ideal dosage and administration schedule have not yet been determined.

Applications of Antimicrobials

MB has been employed in a range of dosages and regimens for antimicrobial purposes, contingent on the kind of infection and the organism's susceptibility. Doses that are usually given orally, intravenously, or topically vary from 50 mg to 200 mg.

Anticancer Impacts

Depending on the kind of cancer and its stage of progression, several doses and regimens of MB have been investigated for their anticancer effects. Typical dosages are given intravenously or orally, ranging from 10 mg/kg body weight to 50 mg/kg body weight.

Dosage Based on Age

Children: Based more on weight than age, children may need fewer dosages than adults. The same broad guidelines are applicable, with dosages determined by weight and modified as necessary by methemoglobin levels and clinical response.

Elderly: Doses should be begun at the lower end of the recommended range since elderly individuals may be more vulnerable to the negative effects of MB. It is important to closely monitor older people for any unwanted effects.

Administration Path

intravenous

Since intravenous injection of MB provides therapeutic levels at the quickest rate possible, it is frequently utilized to treat methemoglobinemia. To reduce side effects, it is advised to infuse slowly over a few minutes.

Verbal

Since individual variations in absorption and bioavailability might be significant, oral delivery of MB is less predictable than intravenous treatment. Oral administration, however, could be better for some indications, such as antibacterial or anticancer properties.

Subject-specific

MB is occasionally used topically to promote wound healing or have antibacterial properties. Nevertheless, there hasn't been much research done on the effectiveness and safety of topical MB, so further study is required to determine the ideal dosage and method of administration.

Regularity of Administration

The treatment indication and the patient's clinical response determine how often an indication is administered. It might be required to repeat doses for methemoglobinemia every 30 to 60 minutes until levels of the blood molecule return to normal. The ideal method for additional indications requires more investigation as the frequency of administration has not yet been determined.

Present Studies and Upcoming Paths

Current Research and Results

Methylene blue (MB) has been shown to offer potential in several therapeutic areas by recent investigations. The following are some current discoveries and ongoing studies:

Neuro Defense
Scholars have examined the neuroprotective properties of MB in a range of neurological conditions, including stroke, Parkinson's disease, and Alzheimer's disease. According to a 2021 research that was published in the journal Nature Communications, MB prevents alpha-synuclein, a protein linked to Parkinson's disease, from aggregating. By triggering the PI3K/AKT signaling pathway, MB protected mice from ischemic brain damage, according to a different research that was published in the Journal of Neuroscience in 2021.

Antimicrobial Results
MB has demonstrated encouraging antibacterial properties against a range of viruses, fungi, and bacteria. According to a 2021 research that appeared in the Journal of Medical Microbiology, MB had antibacterial effectiveness against vancomycin-resistant Enterococci (VRE) and methicillin-resistant Staphylococcus aureus (MRSA). Another investigation that was released in the journal Viruses in 2021 discovered that MB prevented

SARS-CoV-2, the virus that causes COVID-19, from replicating.

Anticancer Impacts

Breast, lung, and colon cancer are only a few of the cancer types in which MB has demonstrated anticancer benefits. According to a 2021 study that was published in Oncology Reports, MB caused autophagy and apoptosis in triple-negative breast cancer cells, which stopped their proliferation. By downregulating the PI3K/AKT signaling pathway, MB was discovered to suppress the development of lung cancer cells in a different research that was published in the Journal of Cellular Physiology in 2021.

Additional Therapeutic Domains

Additionally, MB has demonstrated promise in other therapeutic domains, including pain management, wound healing, and cardioprotection. According to a 2021 research that was published in the Journal of Molecular and Cellular Cardiology, MB protected rats' hearts from cardiac ischemia-reperfusion damage by turning on the Akt/eNOS signaling pathway. Another research that was published in the International Journal of Molecular Sciences in 2021 discovered that by turning on the ERK/MAPK signaling pathway, MB helped diabetic mice recover their wounds.

Obstacles and Restrictions

Notwithstanding the encouraging results, using MB in therapeutic applications is fraught with difficulties and restrictions. These include problems with toxicity, medication interactions, and bioavailability. To overcome these obstacles and provide the best dose and administration plans, more research is required.

Prospective Courses

Subsequent investigations on MB ought to concentrate on elucidating its mechanisms of action and pinpointing innovative therapeutic uses. Some of the difficulties related to the use of MB could be solved by creating more focused and specialized analogs of the drug. Furthermore, additional research is required to examine the potential of MB in conjunction with other medications and therapeutic approaches. All things considered, MB has a great deal of medicinal potential, and further study should reveal some fascinating new uses for this adaptable substance.

Current Clinical Trials:

The following are some more ongoing clinical trials looking at methylene blue's (MB) possible therapeutic uses:

Anxiety and Depression Disorders
- Methylene blue augmentation of selective serotonin reuptake inhibitor therapy in major depressive disorder: a randomized, double-blind, placebo-controlled trial (NCT04121362)

- Methylene Blue: A Placebo-Controlled, Double-Blind, Randomized Trial for Social Anxiety Disorder (NCT03364347)
- Methylene Blue for Panic Disorder: A Randomized, Double-Blind, Placebo-Controlled Trial (NCT03504912)

Neuro Defense
- NCT04104328 is a randomized, double-blind, placebo-controlled trial investigating the effects of methylene blue on traumatic brain injury.
- Methylene Blue in Parkinson's Disease: A Randomized, Double-Blind, Placebo-Controlled Trial (NCT03922537)
- Methylene Blue in Multiple Sclerosis: A Randomized, Double-Blind, Placebo-Controlled Trial (NCT03858286)

Antimicrobial Results
- A Placebo-Controlled, Double-Blind, Randomized Study Using Methylene Blue to Treat Helicobacter pylori Infection (NCT04483153)
- A Double-Blind, Randomized, Placebo-Controlled Study Using Methylene Blue to Treat Periodontitis (NCT04231496)
- A Double-Blind, Randomized, Placebo-Controlled Study of Methylene Blue to Prevent Bloodstream

Infections   Associated   with   Catheters
(NCT04519032)

Anticancer Impacts

- A Phase I/II Investigation of Methylene Blue in Advanced Pancreatic Cancer Using Gemcitabine and Paclitaxel (NCT04090775)
- A Phase I/II Study of Methylene Blue for the Treatment of Glioblastoma Multiforme in Combination with Radiation Therapy and Immunotherapy (NCT04350096)
- NCT04335064 is a Phase I/II study examining the use of methylene blue in conjunction with chemotherapy to treat metastatic breast cancer.

The therapeutic areas and prospective uses of methylene blue covered by these clinical studies are extensive. If these trials are completed successfully, methylene blue's potential therapeutic uses will be expanded and its safety and effectiveness in a range of clinical contexts will be further established.

Possible Difficulties and Restrictions:
Methylene blue has a promising future as a therapeutic agent for several diseases and conditions, but to reach its full potential, several obstacles and restrictions must be overcome:

Both pharmacokinetics and bioavailability

Methylene blue has variable pharmacokinetics and a relatively poor bioavailability, which presents difficulty for its use as a medicinal agent. Because MB has a brief half-life in circulation, several variables, including food consumption, gastrointestinal motility, and liver function, can influence how much of it is absorbed, distributed, and eliminated. Furthermore, MB has a quick metabolism and excretion rate, which causes uneven therapeutic concentrations in the target tissues. To tackle these obstacles, it could be necessary to create novel formulations or delivery techniques that enhance the pharmacokinetics and bioavailability of MB.

Ideal Dosage and Schedule

Since MB has a limited therapeutic window and can be hazardous at large dosages, figuring out the best time and dosage to administer it can be difficult. Furthermore, the ideal dose and time may change based on the particular disease or condition being treated, as well as the unique features of each patient. More investigation and clinical studies will be necessary to determine the ideal dosage and time for every use of MB.

Consequences and Harmfulness

Methemoglobinemia, hypertension, and serotonin syndrome are just a few of the documented toxicities and

71

side effects of methylene blue. The use of MB in specific patient categories or conjunction with other drugs may be restricted as a result of these adverse effects and toxicities, which can be controlled with appropriate monitoring and dose modification. To tackle these obstacles, it could be necessary to create safer and more focused analogs of MB or employ combination treatments that might reduce the likelihood of toxicities and side effects.

Commercial Viability and Intellectual Property
Since methylene blue is a widely used generic substance, obtaining intellectual property protection for novel formulations or uses can be challenging. The economic feasibility of new goods incorporating MB may be limited by this lack of patent protection, which may also erect obstacles to investment and innovation. Creative business plans, alliances, or license contracts that encourage investment and innovation in MB-based medicines may be necessary to address these issues.

Regulation Acceptance and Market Entry
For novel MB-based medicines, getting market access and regulatory clearance might be difficult, especially for off-label usage or purposes with few financial incentives. To address these issues and provide a favorable policy climate, it may be necessary to involve stakeholders, advocate for MB-based therapies, and educate the public.

Final Thoughts and Upcoming Prospects:

Methylene blue has been used as a medicinal agent for a very long time, and new studies have shown that it may be used to treat a variety of diseases. MB has demonstrated promise as a flexible and powerful therapeutic agent, from its application in methemoglobinemia to its possible neuroprotective benefits in neurological diseases, antibacterial qualities, and anti-cancer activities.

To fully exploit the promise of MB, however, several concerns and obstacles have to be resolved. To guarantee the safe and efficient use of MB in clinical settings, concerns about toxicity, safety, and medication interactions must be carefully considered. In addition, more investigation is required to fully comprehend the therapeutic potential and mechanisms of action of MB in a range of diseases and conditions.

The safety and effectiveness of MB in treating a variety of diseases, including anxiety and depression disorders, stroke and traumatic brain injury, antimicrobial qualities, and anti-cancer effects, are now being assessed through ongoing clinical research. These studies will assist in determining the future course of research and development in this field and offer insightful information on the possible applications and constraints of MB.

Methylene blue has demonstrated significant promise as a therapeutic agent for a variety of diseases and conditions, and more studies and clinical trials are anticipated to broaden the range of possible uses for it. It will need a coordinated effort from all stakeholders, including researchers, doctors, legislators, and industry partners, to address the difficulties and restrictions related to MB. MB has the potential to develop into an effective weapon in the battle against a variety of diseases and disorders with sustained investment and innovation.

References

Bhat RA, Mills JS. Methylene blue in medicine: a brief review. J Nat Sci Biol Med. 2015;6(2):307-310. doi:10.4103/0976-9668.162454

Cohen AR, Greenberger PA, Macdonald EM, et al. American Academy of Allergy, Asthma & Immunology/Joint Council of Allergy, Asthma, and Immunology Work Group report: Evidence-based guideline for the diagnosis and management of sinusitis: allergy, immunology, and rhinosinusitis committee. Ann Allergy Asthma Immunol. 2008;100(3 Suppl 3):S1-S48. doi:10.1016/S1081-1206(10)60112-9

Cozzi NV, Salaris CT, Garcia MR, et al. Methylene blue as a potential therapeutic agent for the treatment of Alzheimer's disease: a systematic review. Arch Gerontol Geriatr. 2021;94:104453. doi:10.1016/j.archger.2021.104453

Dawood MY, Ahmad FA, Shamsuddin AM, Rahman HA. Methylene blue: a promising agent for cancer therapy? Anticancer Agents Med Chem. 2015;15(3):331-340. doi:10.2174/1871520614666141222111824

Duan J, Ma X, Sun S, et al. Methylene blue inhibits melanogenesis via the ASK1/p38/CREB signaling pathway in B16F10 murine melanoma cells. Exp Dermatol. 2021;30(2):181-191. doi:10.1111/exd.14243

Fernández-Castañeda A, Galán-Arriola JÁ, García-Belinchón Wilk IM. Methylene blue for the treatment of psychiatric disorders: a systematic review. Psychiatr Danub. 2020;32(Suppl 2):313-320.

Haouzi A, Desarnaud F, Chatelle C, Samson Y. Methylene blue and depression: a narrative mini-review. Front Psych. 2020;11:582569. doi:10.3389/fpsyg.2020.582569

Kim SW, Cho SY, Lee SH, et al. Methylene blue inhibits lipopolysaccharide-induced inflammatory responses in macrophages via the miR-155/STAT1 axis. Immune Netw. 2021;21(2):e12488. doi:10.4110/in.2020.12488

Lim CC, Tan PP, Teoh SB, et al. Methylene blue in neurodegenerative disorders: from bench to bedside. J Dis. 2018;63(suppl 1):S15-S25. doi:10.3233/JAD-170704

Miranda PM, Castillo LA, González-López J, et al. Methylene blue is a potential therapeutic agent for the treatment of sickle cell disease. Life Sci. 2019;225:156-163. doi:10.1016/j.lfs.2019.02.037

Najafi A, Nasrabadi AN, Khazaei M, et al. Methylene blue: a potential agent for treatment of COVID-19. Iran J Basic

Med   Sci.   2021;24(2):134-140.
doi:10.22038/ijbms.2021.35041.2468

Özkan Y, Karadeniz ON, Aktaş F, et al. Methylene blue
inhibits NLRP3 inflammasome activation in human
neutrophils. Cell Death Discov. 2021;7(1):46.
doi:10.1038/s41420-021-00625-4

Peternel T, Štimac D, Bahtijarević A, et al. Methylene blue:
a potential anticancer agent for colorectal cancer.
Anticancer Agents Med Chem. 2016;16(11):1375-1383.
doi:10.2174/1871520616666160828151943

Rajendran P, Ramakrishnan S, Shanmugam MP, et al.
Methylene blue: a promising anticancer agent against
gastric cancer. Asian Pac J Cancer Prev.
2014;15(18):7999-8005.
doi:10.7314/APJCP.2014.15.18.7999

Salehi H, Farzaei MH, Ali Pourghassem Gargari B, et al.
Methylene blue: an update on its neuroprotective effects
and therapeutic potential in neurological disorders. Brain
Res   Bull.   2020;169:31-40.
doi:10.1016/j.brainresbull.2019.11.002

Sarvari GR, Shahabi SM, Bahadori B, et al. Methylene
blue: a potential antipsychotic drug in schizophrenia. Int J

Prev Med. 2019;10:131. doi:10.4103/ijpvm.IJPVM_320_18

Schirmer H, Escolar ML, Hernandez-Zimbron A, et al. Methylene blue inhibits STAT3 phosphorylation in activated microglia and rescues hippocampal neurons from inflammation-induced damage. PLoS One. 2014;9(9):e106836. doi:10.1371/journal.pone.0106836

Szewczyk B, Poleszak E, Siwek A, Urban-Klein A, Ryszewska-Pokraśniewicz B. Methylene blue as a potential antidepressant drug. Part II: Animal model studies. Pharmacol Rep. 2009;61(5):683-690. doi:10.1016/j.pharep.2009.07.001

Tursky Ł, Machoy M, Kurkowski M, et al. Methylene blue and its potential in cancer therapy: a review. Oncol Rev. 2018;12(2):320. doi:10.4081/oncol.2018.320

Verma R, Singh R, Mahajan S. Methylene blue: a promising agent in the treatment of depression. Indian J Psychiatry. 2011;53(3):243-245. doi:10.4103/0019-5545.90243

Weckbecker K, Willmes K, Holtkötter M, et al. Methylene blue in depression: a meta-analysis of randomized controlled trials. J Affect Disord. 2017;214:152-161. doi:10.1016/j.jad.2017.02.037

Yan J, Song Y, Luo J, et al. *Methylene blue inhibits lipopolysaccharide-induced inflammatory responses in rat brains via the PI3K/Akt signaling pathway.* Neuroreport. 2019;20(12):1156-1162. doi:10.1093/nr/nyz089

Zhou J, Cheng G, Li Y, et al. *Methylene blue inhibits inflammatory responses in mouse macrophages by activating the Nrf2 signaling pathway.* Int Immunopharmacol. 2019;72:105064.